"There is no magic pill or formula for beating back nicotine addiction," Dr. Brunswick said. "However, with a better understanding of why you smoke and the different tools you can use to control the urge to light up, you can stop being a slave to your cigarettes."

—*Jane E. Brody*
The New York Times

Quit smoking—easier said than done? Using simple, proven method this little book has everything a smoker needs to quit. Doctors advise patients to quit smoking all the time; if this book were given with that advice, there would be fewer smokers and far more ex-smokers in the world today. I encourage *Can't Quit? Bullsh*t!* for all smokers who want to be free of this addiction."

—*Frank Verloin deGruy III, MD,*
Professor and Chair, Department of Family
Medicine, University of Colorado School
of Medicine

A very practical guide to the task of quitting tobacco. I recommend that doctors, dentists, and caregivers hand one out to anyone with nicotine addiction. I heartily endorse this new book for any smoker trying to break the habit.

—*Alan Calhoun, MD*
Director, University Health Service
University of Massachusetts, Amherst

Richard Brunswick, MD

Can't Quit?
Bullsh*t!

You *Can* Stop Smoking

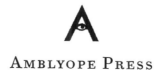

AMBLYOPE PRESS

Publication date January 2013

Text copyright ©2013 Richard Brunswick

Illustrations ©2013 Elena Betke-Brunswick

All rights reserved

Published by Amblyope Press
Northampton, Massachusetts

Designed by Hans Teensma
Produced by Impress
Williamsburg, Massachusetts

Brunswick, Richard, 1952-
   Can't quit? bullsh*t! : you can stop smoking /
Richard Brunswick.
   p. cm.
   LCCN 2012918575
   ISBN 978-0-9884372-0-3

   1. Nicotine addiction–Treatment. 2. Smoking
cessation. 3. Smoking–Health aspects.   I. Title.
II. Title: Can't quit? bullshit!

RC567.B78 2012   616.86'506
                        QBI12-600209

Printed in the U.S.A.

10 9 8 7 6 5 4 3 2 1

It's not because things are difficult that we do not dare; it is because we do not dare that they are difficult.

—*Seneca*

Roman dramatist, philospher, and politician (5 BC – 65 AD)

LEGAL NOTICE

This book is meant to give helpful information on stopping smoking. Neither the author nor the publisher is your personal doctor giving you professional medical care or counseling to diagnose or treat any condition, even smoking/nicotine addiction. You should see your doctor about stopping smoking and about the advice in this book.

The author and publisher have made great effort to make this accurate. Even so, it may have mistakes in writing, printing, or content. It should be used as a general guide only. What it says is current up to the date of publication and is the author's personal opinion only.

The author and publisher shall have neither liability nor responsibility to any person or entity with respect to any loss or damages caused or alleged to be caused, directly or indirectly, by the information in this book. The author and publisher are not responsible for the content of any website; the safety and effectiveness of any products, devices, or medications; or the advice and representations of any companies or organizations named in this book.

TABLE OF CONTENTS

INTRODUCTION

You are not the problem. Addiction is the problem. You can overcome your addiction to smoking. I became a family doctor in 1984, and since then I've helped many smokers quit.

Rewards from stopping smoking include a healthier life and family, saved money, better sex, and knowing you can take on challenges—such as quitting—and succeed. Even though quitting smoking is the best thing you can do for your health, it meets a need, so you keep lighting up. As we'll see, there are better ways to meet those needs.

As a doctor I've taken care of many smokers with breathing and other health problems, and I want to help people avoid trouble down the road. Due to difficult-to-control asthma, I've had major breathing problems of my own. That's why I'm passionate about this topic, and that's why I wrote this book.

Some of the people I've helped smoked five cigarettes a day; others smoked three packs. They've been of all ages, poor and well-off, and from many different countries. Quite a few of them had tried to quit before but were still smoking when they first came to see me. I've written this book to share with you what I know about how they overcame their addiction to cigarettes.

Unfortunately, there is no magic pill or formula for beating back nicotine addiction. However, with a better understanding of why you smoke and the different tools you can use to control the urge to light up, you can stop being a slave to your cigarettes.

The tobacco companies want to sell more cigarettes to make more money. They design their product in ways that make it easy to start and hard to stop. If you believe you can't stop, you keep smoking—and they make more money. Multiply that by everyone who's smoking, and it's a lot of money. They win; you lose.

What if quitting isn't so hard to do? Think about it: you probably know people who have quit, yet you still think you can't. You can do it too. If you've lived long enough to read this book, you've done harder things in your life.

You'd probably like to stop smoking if you thought you could do it. I wrote this book to give you a way to make it happen. You'll meet Emily and Ben, a couple who quit together using my approach. You'll also meet some of the other patients I've met over the years. Their names and the stories I tell about them are disguised but based on experiences with my patients over many years.

There are five chapters to this short book. The first, "Before You Quit," prepares you for the challenge ahead. The second, "Ten Steps to Quitting," provides useful and clear steps to follow to become a nonsmoker. The third, "After You Quit," will help you keep from starting up again. A brief chapter follows that addresses those of you who want to stop smoking, stay healthy, and stay on nicotine. This material may save your life. The book ends with additional information on stopping-smoking resources, medicines that make stopping smoking easier, and lowering tobacco's harm. I suggest you read the whole book before you begin the steps to quitting.

Then go back and use the steps.

If you read this book and do what it says, you *can* quit smoking and have a much healthier, longer life. I've seen many people stop smoking using my method. There are now more ex-smokers in the United States than there are active smokers. Wherever you live, you can be one of the ex-smokers too.

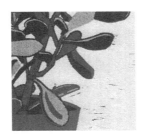

JADE

I

BEFORE
YOU
QUIT

*You began smoking
without planning to be
smoking years later.*

Addiction

EMILY began smoking when she was seventeen. Ben started when he went to work in construction, at age nineteen. Although they each began by having two or three cigarettes a day, by the time they were in their late twenties, both smoked a little over a pack a day. What began as a way to feel pleasure became, with continued smoking, a way to avoid the discomfort of nicotine withdrawal.

Ben and Emily, like many people I've seen over the years, told me they wouldn't have started smoking if they'd known what it was all about. It's likely you began smoking with no plan to be smoking years later. Addiction sneaked up on you. Understanding how that happens will help you understand how to end it.

The reason nicotine hooks you is

because it reaches the brain so quickly. It gives you a small energy boost (and relaxes you at the same time), improves your mood, and sharpens your focus. A lot of that is relief from the tired, down feelings of withdrawal from your last cigarette. After each cigarette, withdrawal starts again. You have another cigarette to feed the habit, and before you know it, you've smoked another pack.

Being addicted is about needing more nicotine. It's a drug habit. Smoking, like any habit, has three parts: **triggers**, **routines**, and **rewards**.[1] Here's what you need to know about them to break the habit.

Triggers. Triggers are what lead you to want to light up so that you get the rewards that nicotine gives you. Your brain is changed by nicotine, and it wants more! Triggers usually relate to a time of day, a place, mood, or other people.[2] Seeing, smelling, or tasting also work as triggers: for example, seeing an ashtray, smelling cigarette smoke, or tasting something that reminds you of your brand's flavor. Triggers also lead to slip-ups—the smoke you didn't plan to have after you quit. Some common smoking triggers are:

- Waking up (time)

- Feeling helpless, hopeless, sad, angry, or bored (mood)

- Taking a work break (time)

- Being with smokers (people)

- Being in a bar or having a drink (place)

- Traveling to and from work (place)

- Having a meal or coffee and dessert (time)

Routines. Routines are the smoking patterns in your life, such as the hand you use to hold the cigarette or lighter or where you keep your pack. Routines are also tied to events in your life. For example, if you always light up in your car on the way to work and stop to buy more cigarettes at the same store every time, it's part of your smoking routine. Sticking to new routines that don't include smoking is a big part of beating the habit.

Rewards. The main reward from smoking is avoidance of nicotine withdrawal. Withdrawal causes nervousness and irritability. Having more nicotine relieves this stress and gives more energy, better focus, and relief once you light up. Your reward may be taking a break, time out from stress, or keeping weight off. There are plenty of other rewards, such as feeling cool, grown up, or part of a group of people who smoke. Every smoker has a favorite reward. Think about what yours is.

Emily had her first cigarette of the day on her way to work so she wouldn't smoke indoors around her children. She smoked whenever she spent time with her mom or best friend, both of whom were smokers too. She lit up after arguments with Ben. She also smoked during work breaks and even when out for a walk during her lunch break.

Ben, on the other hand, lit up as soon as he got out of bed in the morning, after sex, on work breaks, and after meals. Sometimes Ben smoked when he needed more energy at work.

They both smoked with friends when they went out to a bar or over to their best friends' home. They smoked to relax and when they were bored, to help time pass, or to improve mood.

By knowing and avoiding your triggers, by changing your routines, by going through withdrawal in a way that doesn't feel so bad, and by finding new rewards without lighting up you can stop for good. Keep reading, and you'll learn how.

The risk of a heart attack
from smoking falls off quickly
once you've quit.

Withdrawal

EMILY expected withdrawal to be really awful. To her surprise it was mild and easy to handle. Ben, however, found it hard. Withdrawal isn't the same for everyone. Some find going through it really easy, some say it is hard but not bad, and others find it really difficult. In my practice I've had many more people say it was much easier than they expected it to be, but almost all thought it would be bad. Because of fear that it would be awful, many had never even tried to quit even though they wanted to stop.

Withdrawal is part of getting better! You may feel lousy, but the feeling is short-term, and the result is good for you. Because all the poisons in tobacco smoke begin to leave your body the day you quit, your body begins to heal quickly. The heart attack risk from smoking goes way down in a matter of days.

When you don't smoke for a few hours or overnight, that lousy feeling and strong need for a smoke are the start of withdrawal. That's why Ben lit up first thing each morning. The longer you go without a smoke, the worse the feeling gets until withdrawal is over.

Think of withdrawal the same way you think of a cold—you get over it. The worst of withdrawal is over in four days, and almost all the rest of it is gone within a month. The second day is usually the hardest. The hardest part for some is low mood. Low mood can last, but I'll tell you what to do about that too.

The urges to smoke, also called cravings, lead to starting up again. Cravings are difficult for many, but they're not the same thing as withdrawal, which lasts only days to weeks. The urges go on far longer. You'll learn how to cope with cravings in the steps that follow.

In addition to using nicotine patches, gum, or lozenges to lessen withdrawal, here are other things you can do while you're waiting for it to pass.

Symptom	What to do
Cough	Sip water; suck on cough drops
Feeling grumpy, stressed	Drink tea; go for walks; call a friend; take ten slow, deep breaths
Feeling tired, less focused	Exercise; relax; cut back on tasks
Constipation, mouth sores	Drink more water; eat grains, fruit, and vegetables
Headaches, light-headedness	Place cool compress on forehead; take acetaminophen or ibuprofen

Smoking causes trouble. Withdrawal will probably be less trouble than you think. By quitting, you'll spare yourself a lot more trouble from ill health later.

The average smoker shortens his or her life by ten years.

Why are you smoking?
Why are you quitting?

EMILY and Ben both smoked to relax. Ben smoked at work for the energy boost and to take a break.

What are your reasons for smoking? People smoke for many reasons, but for each smoker, smoking fills a need. Usually that need is to feel better. Many smokers say they feel more relaxed after a smoke and that they have more energy. There's nothing wrong with feeling better; it's a good thing. Unfortunately, smoking to feel better in the short term comes with the long-term price of ill health. You can feel better and live longer if you don't smoke.

Smoking causes heart attacks, lung and other cancers, strokes, lung trouble, erectile dysfunction (E.D.), lower pregnancy rates and low-birth-weight babies, and many other problems. Ben was interested in quitting because a doctor told one of his friends that his E.D. was caused by smoking. He went to the Internet and learned that smoking is a common cause of E.D.

The average smoker shortens his life by ten years compared to a nonsmoker. These are some of the long-term prices you pay for smoking. You're kidding yourself if you believe that illness and an early death from smoking won't happen to you. You probably already know the risks, whether right up front or in the back of your mind, and may feel bad that you're still smoking.

What are your reasons for quitting? The high costs in money and health are two common ones, but they're not the only reasons people have for stopping. Emily and Ben decided to quit when they realized that together they were spending over $5,000 a year on cigarettes. By stopping they'd stay fit, have more energy, and keep enjoying sex for many more years. Write your reasons for quitting, put them where you can see them, and read them every day.

You won't fall apart if you don't light up. Lighting up doesn't solve problems, but it does cause new ones.

Tried to quit before? Do it a different way this time.

THE FIRST TIME Ben tried to quit he chose a date, went "cold turkey," and lasted just three days without a smoke. Going cold turkey means quitting smoking all at once. One minute you're a smoker, the next minute you're an ex-smoker. The next time Ben quit he lasted two weeks before he started smoking again. This time he made plans, did some preparing, got help, and used nicotine patches. Emily's story was similar, but she didn't use a medicine.

It's great that you plan to quit, but take a good look at how you go about it so you stop for good. If you've quit and started up before, you don't want to stop and start up all over again.

Do things differently this time! Answer the following questions, paying attention to what you think went wrong last time so you can address that problem this time around.

- What was the hardest part about quitting last time?

- Did I have any help, such as a telephone quit line or online support program?

- Did I have a quit buddy, someone to call for help to keep me smoke-free?

- Was I sad or anxious, and before quitting did I consider dealing with my mood problems?

- Did I know my triggers?

- Did I spend my free time with smokers and/or out drinking?

- Did I change my routines when I quit?

- Did I really decide to quit, or was I just making believe I would quit?

- Did I go back to smoking after the first slip-up? If so, why? Did I plan for slip-ups and know how to deal with them?

- Did I think about taking a drug for a few months to help with withdrawal?

- Did I have a plan for coping with urges to smoke?

Emily and Ben had each tried to quit two or three times before. They did eventually quit. You also have the power to quit, just as they did.

You know people
who have quit.
You can do it too.

Be honest with yourself

QUITTING is hard enough. It's time to quit only if you're ready and serious about doing it. What I saw as a doctor boils down to this: if you've tried to cut down and have a date to stop, you're probably ready, with a little preparation, to quit. If you've thought about quitting within the next three months or so, you are nearly ready. If you never think about stopping and have no plans to do so, you aren't ready. If you're not ready to stop, wait until you are. If you're reading this book, you're probably ready, but you're more likely to be successful if you set up a plan to do it.

Do you have to stop drinking or using drugs in order to give up smoking? Maybe or maybe not: you may need help figuring that out. Drinking, drug use, and smoking often go together. If you are going to quit, cutting down or stopping drinking or drug use does help you stay tobacco-free. If you're drinking or using drugs too much, as many do, and can't stop or cut back, get help from your doctor or use the resources at the end of the book. If you drink and smoke, stopping one doesn't prevent you from stopping the other. Some experts suggest you tackle one addiction at a time, others say it's best to stop both as soon as you're ready.

When Ben and Emily quit, they had little trouble staying smoke-free all during the work week, but on weekends, when out with friends, they'd start smoking again while having a few beers. They changed their weekend routines, cut back on their drinking, and found that doing so really helped them quit.

Sadness that lasts (depression) and too much worry (anxiety) are common problems that don't come only from nicotine withdrawal. Many people suffer with these conditions. If you have little joy in life and feel hopeless, tired, and lacking in energy, you may be depressed. If you worry a lot, are always on edge, and are fearful of what may come next, you may be anxious. Getting help for too much sadness, stress, and anxiety not only makes life more enjoyable but also makes quitting much easier.

You might be scared of quitting. If you think you won't be able to cope with day-to-day life without smoking and that life's stresses will be too hard to handle, you're wrong! You won't fall apart if you don't light up, but it helps to have another way to handle the stress without lighting up.

Feeling angry, helpless, or bored also may lead you to light up. That's why Emily lit up whenever she and Ben argued. When you have strong emotions, recognize them, and don't light up. Lighting up doesn't solve problems, but it does cause new ones. Once Emily realized she could be angry at Ben and not light up, she found it easy to do.

Take a look at your readiness to stop, your emotions, and your alcohol and drug use. Are you ready? If so, go for it!

You'd have to gain over eighty pounds to cause as much harm to yourself as you do by smoking.

Don't diet—just quit

EMILY had tried to quit twice before her latest try. Each time, after gaining five pounds, she started smoking again and lost the five pounds within a month. When she finally quit, she gained eight pounds in three months. One year later she had lost five of them and still wasn't smoking.

Many people worry about gaining weight when they quit, and it keeps them from quitting. The bad news is it's true—most smokers do gain five to twelve pounds when quitting because nicotine lowers appetite and affects how the body handles calories. The good news is that compared to smoking, a little weight gain is much better for your overall health. You'd have to gain over eighty pounds to cause as much harm to yourself as you do by smoking.[3]

Take on one challenge at a time. When you are quitting, accept that some weight gain will likely happen and try not to worry about it. If you focus on both not gaining and not smoking, you may end up still smoking and gaining.

Here are some tips on weight gain and quitting:

- Quit smoking first.

- If you gain some weight, accept it. Don't go back to smoking to lose it.

- When you quit, if at all possible, increase your walking to thirty to sixty minutes a day.

- Chew sugar-free gum when you have an urge to smoke.

- Snack on things like pretzels, fresh fruit, raw vegetables, and popcorn without butter or oil.

- Drink plenty of water.

After you've been smoke-free for six or twelve months, start to work on losing any gained weight.[4] This can be your next challenge.

Consider taking a medicine called bupropion, also known by the name Zyban, to help you quit smoking. It will also help you keep weight off.

When Emily did quit, she did all those things except take bupropion. She quit, and she weighs three pounds more than before she quit. She's happy, and with the money she's saving by not buying cigarettes she's looking forward to some really nice vacations and an extra ten years of life!

She took these healthy steps. You can take them too.

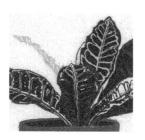

CROTON

2

TEN
STEPS TO
QUITTING

You don't "have to"
light up and you don't
"need" a smoke.

Step 1
Commit to quit

IF YOU THINK it's impossible to quit—that it's hopeless to even try—you're wrong. You've met people who've stopped smoking. How did they do it? For Ben and Emily and every other ex-smoker, it began with the decision to stop.

Quitting doesn't start when you decide to try to quit; it happens when you decide to be an ex-smoker.

This may be a surprise to you: most smokers don't quit on their first few tries. Studies show that people with a history of failed attempts at quitting are more likely to stop for good compared with those who've never even tried before. Think of those earlier tries as steps on the way to being smoke-free. They are what you needed to learn in order to stop for good.

When you are ready to quit, commit yourself to it by writing down your goal. Tell friends and family that you are stopping smoking. This makes you responsible for your actions and can help boost your efforts to stay smoke-free. Tell yourself and others that you have decided to free yourself of tobacco and that you have quit. But if you think you'll do better by not telling anyone, that's fine too.

Don't try to quit. Instead, just quit. Willpower has little to do with quitting. A plan with steps will help you quit.

Reading this book doesn't make you quit; you make yourself quit by following the book's directions. You are addicted, but you still can choose to be free of your addiction. You don't "have to" light up and you don't "need" a smoke.

Smoking isn't your "friend."
Your friends don't poison you.

Step 2

Say good-bye to smoking and hello to your future

B EN CAME to see me after one of his earlier quit attempts, when he started up again after two weeks without a smoke. He said, "If only I wasn't a loser, I could quit."

I told him, "Ben, you're not a loser, you're a nicotine addict."

If you feel the way Ben did, you need to accept that you are not the problem, but that nicotine addiction has got hold of you. It won't let go unless you fight for your freedom. You need to get ready for that fight.

Writing a "Dear John" letter is part of that fight. The usual Dear John letter is written to break up a dating relationship— you're breaking up with smoking! The letter could say what smoking has meant to you and why the relationship is over. You could write about what you wish for in the future. Doing this will firm up your plan to quit.

Here's what Emily wrote to smoking.

Dear stinky habit,

I'm writing to tell you a few things and to say good-bye. You did make me feel more awake and alive, gave me something to do, and helped me feel a part of the action. You gave me a break from stress.

I've thought about what you want for me and what I want instead. I don't want the embarrassment of being a smoker, the smelly clothes, or your poison. I know you'll make me short of breath and maybe give me cancer or heart trouble. You'll cost me lots of money, and you're really not helping me control my weight.

I'm taking this step as someone who can get things done. I can take care of business now.

When I'm a nonsmoker, my kids will be less likely to start smoking or miss school with colds. With the money I save by not smoking, we'll be able to do things we've always talked about. We'll save and maybe buy a home or

*take a vacation. I'll be far more likely to enjoy
my family when older.*

*For a long time I didn't think I'd ever quit.
Uncle Ed wouldn't be surprised to know I'm
really quitting. He always believed in me.
Though I've done other hard things, like my job
and being a good mom, I thought I'd never stop.
It won't be so hard. I'm looking forward to this
and other challenges.*

*By quitting I'm becoming my own best
friend.* [5]

Emily

There's no right way to write a letter. Your
story is your own.

Though it may seem hokey, don't skip
this step. Trust the process. Take your
time to think about why you are saying
good-bye and how you'll be different once
you quit. Honor your past and your future
with a letter.

You did not create this problem, but you
are the one who must fix it.

There are more ex-smokers than smokers in the United States.

STEP 3
Outwit tobacco's tricks

DON'T BELIEVE everything you think! It really helps you quit if you look at beliefs you may have developed as your addiction took hold. If you find you have any of the following thoughts, notice them and correct your thinking.[6] Challenge your thoughts. Tell yourself what is really true.

FALSE	TRUE
A cigarette is a reward.	A cigarette is a poison.
Health troubles from smoking won't happen to me.	The odds are that they will happen to me if I continue smoking.
I can't have fun without smoking.	I can and did have fun before I began smoking.
Quitting will make me sick.	Smoking makes me sick.
People will think I'm a failure if I can't quit.	People know that quitting isn't easy.
Smoking relieves stress.	It relieves withdrawal, which is stressful. Taking breaks and slow, deep breathing relieve stress.

FALSE	TRUE
It will be like losing my best friend.	Smoking isn't my "friend." Friends don't poison me!
I'll gain a ton of weight.	I'll probably gain five to ten pounds. I can lose them later.
I really like smoking.	Do I? Or is it the break and relaxation I like? I can take a break and relax without the smoke.
It's hopeless to try to quit; I'll never do it.	It's not. Many have quit. I can do it too.

There are more ex-smokers in the United States than smokers! Examine your own thinking and fix what's not true. Add untrue thoughts to this list and read it each day.

*Addiction won't let go
of you unless you
fight for your freedom.*

Step 4
Track your triggers, then rework the reward

EMILY REALIZED she lit up whenever she talked with her best friend. Ben would grab a coffee and sit outside after lunch for a smoke. Emily smoked when upset or bored. They didn't decide to smoke at those times. Most smokers light up on autopilot, without awareness. That may be what you do too.

To become more aware of each smoke so that you're not on autopilot, here are two simple things you can do: change brands, and change hands to the one you don't usually use to smoke. Instead of your usual brand, switch to a brand you know you don't like.[7] If you use your right hand to hold the cigarette, switch to your left from now on.[8] Making these simple changes will take you off autopilot and give you a moment to consider whether you'll have the smoke or skip it. You'll also have a chance to think about other ways to relax or to sharpen your focus, such as taking deep breaths, taking a break, or doing some exercises.

Take five minutes to write down your triggers for smoking, buying cigarettes, or thinking about smoking. Think about when you smoke. Do you light up when

- getting out of bed to start your day?

- driving to work or school?

- feeling bored or stressed?

- having alcohol, coffee, or a meal?

- smelling or seeing cigarette smoke?

- spending time with particular people?

I've had lots of patients who were able to be smoke-free all week until Friday or Saturday night. Then they'd be drinking with friends and would light up. Here's why: three of the most common situations that trigger smoking are drinking alcohol, being around other smokers, and being in a bad mood. If several of these conditions occur at the same time, it becomes very difficult to stay smoke-free. Be aware of these three triggers and plan to avoid them.[9] Cut your time around other triggers too.

Pay attention to triggers and change the routines that follow them. This will help you learn to cope without the smoke.

When you have a strong urge for a smoke, use any or all of the four Ds to get past it: **delay**, as it'll pass quickly; take five or ten slow, **deep breaths**; **drink** some water in sips; and **distract** yourself to take your mind off smoking.[10]

Develop a new reward similar to what you believe you get from smoking. You could use a piece of nicotine gum or take ten deep breaths and imagine healthier lungs. You can do some quick exercises for good health or take a short break from a hectic day.[11] Find a reward that will work for you.

Tell yourself and everyone else, "No, I don't smoke anymore," and let the reward be your sense of accomplishment.

You are not the problem.
Addiction is the problem.

STEP 5
Retrain your brain with new routines

EMILY always smoked on the way to work. Ben and Emily spent Friday nights at a bar with buddies. They told me that changing routines really helped.

Why will new routines help with quitting? Smoking has patterns or routines: the when, where, and how of smoking. As mentioned earlier, when you light up, where you keep your pack, where you buy cigarettes, and which hand you use to hold a lighter are all part of your habit. Your brain learned these patterns. When you change them, your brain develops new patterns after several days or weeks, ones that don't include smoking. Take a few minutes to write down your old smoking routines and for each one, plan a new routine that doesn't include smoking.

Write down your usual routines and the changes you'll make. Here are some examples.[12]

OLD ROUTINE	NEW ROUTINE
Wake up, turn on coffeemaker, smoke and have coffee, head to work	Wake up, shower, take coffee in a travel mug in the now no-smoking car
Dinner, smoke, do dishes	Dinner, go for a walk or play with the kids outdoors, do dishes
Drive to work, passing by the store where you buy smokes	Change your route so you don't pass the store; carpool with a nonsmoker in a no-smoking car

Old routine	New routine
Saturday night on a date at the bar with smoking friends	Saturday night at the movies with friends or drinks in your or a friend's no-smoking home
Smoke with a friend on a nearby park bench	Meet friend at a new place or for a walk and agree neither will smoke

Keeping your hands busy in ways other than smoking is a necessary routine change. You get the cigarette out of the pack, you light it, you bring it back and forth to your mouth, then to an ashtray, and you put it out. This is all part of the addiction. Plan how you'll use your hands once you've stopped. It doesn't matter whether it's taking up a new hobby, doing puzzles, texting or emailing, playing computer or cell phone games, making art, playing cards, doing crafts, or whatever, as long as your hands stay busy.

When you first stop, and for several months after, any way you can find to keep your hands busy will help keep you from smoking. Staying busy with exercise, walking, cooking, reading, and other activities will also help you to stay smoke-free. Your mouth also needs to learn routines other than smoking. Ask yourself what you can do with your mouth other than smoking until you are free of cravings. I've listed some coping methods on page 26 in the section "Don't diet—just quit."

When an urge to smoke strikes, what you do to keep your hands and mouth busy is up to you. You could have a new routine such as sipping water, carrying something small in each hand, popping a sugarless candy in your mouth, or going for a short walk. You can also use the four Ds, discussed in the previous step: delay, deep breaths, drink, distract. Do the stress-relieving activities described on pages 79 to 81. These actions will take away the urge to smoke and will help retrain your brain.

Knowing your old routines and replacing them with new ones that don't include smoking is one of the best things you can do to quit. Tell yourself that your hands and mouth have a new job: keeping you healthy.

Ask your friends who smoke
not to smoke around you,
especially indoors, and
never to offer you a cigarette.

STEP 6

The three Gs— get help, get a buddy, and go public

STOPPING SMOKING isn't something you must do alone. Although you might smoke alone, most people smoke in relation to others. Following this step makes quitting easier.

Get help. Scientists have studied how people quit and what works. They've found that those who get help are the most likely to stop and to remain smoke-free one year later.

What type of help? It's best to call a toll-free telephone quit support line such as 1-800-QUIT-NOW (1-800-784-8669). These professional quit-line services are proven effective, can advise you about helpful quitting and coping methods and medications, and many provide a starting pack of medications at no charge. An online support program such as Smokefree.gov (www.smokefree.gov) gives you access to advice, information, and other quitters twenty-four hours a day, seven days a week. You can also try a quit-smoking group. Groups such as those offered by the American Heart Association, American Lung Association, or American Cancer Society may also be helpful. You'll find contact telephone numbers and web addresses in the Resources section at the end of the book.

Before your quit date, visit your doctor or nurse to discuss quitting. A healthcare professional can help you cope with withdrawal and smoking urges and will tell you about medications to help you stop. It's a good idea to follow up with the doctor or nurse about five days after stopping. You'll know that someone besides you thinks quitting is very, very important.

Emily and Ben went to see their doctor together. They got some handouts on quitting. Ben decided to use a medicine to help him quit. Emily, who didn't smoke as much as Ben, decided against using a medicine. They both called and used telephone quit lines. Emily joined a support group at work for people who were quitting.

Get a buddy. Next, get a quit buddy. A friend can really help when a strong urge to smoke strikes. Your buddy will be your go-to person who has agreed to support your quitting 100 percent. Choose someone you can trust, someone who can cheer you on and cheer you up! This person has already quit or has also, like you, decided to live smoke-free.

Especially during the first week, and through the next full year, your buddy will be the lifeline who you can call if you really feel the urge to smoke and are worried you'll give in. Online quitting services and phone quit lines can also be very helpful for coping with cravings, and help is available 24/7.

Your buddy needs to agree to remind you that urges pass and that most last only a few minutes. A quit buddy is someone who doesn't judge or try to control you. He or she should be a good listener who can help you figure out what to do until the urge passes.

Go public. Next tell your family, friends, and other key people you know that you've quit and ask for their support. Most people know that quitting isn't easy and will want to help you. Have little contact with anyone who doesn't want to help with what's best for you.

There's a saying that 80 percent of success is based on just showing up. If so, then showing up in public as an ex-smoker is part of being one. Some don't want to let others know in case they keep smoking. If you tell everybody you have quit and then aren't able to do it, you don't have to feel shame. Instead you can say, "I didn't quit this time, but I'm planning to try again. I hear that most smokers need a few tries until they quit. I haven't given up. I'll quit again soon."

Emily and Ben asked family and friends to help them avoid triggers and to support the changes they were making. You can ask your family and friends for the same help:

- Ask your friends who smoke not to smoke around you, especially indoors, and never to offer you a cigarette.

- Arrange to meet at places that don't allow smoking.

- Let them know that you are likely to be a bit grumpy for a while and not to take it personally.

- Thank them for helping you on your mission.

Tell yourself that your real friends want you to stay healthy. From now on you're showing up as an ex-smoker.

*Why not use a medication
for three months to prevent
a heart attack, stroke,
or cancer?*

Step 7
Consider medication

You'd probably take a drug to treat high blood pressure, an allergy, or strep throat. Why not take one for a few months if it will help you stop smoking and prevent a heart attack, stroke, or cancer? By doing so you double your chances of being smoke-free one year later. If you add medicines to the other supports you put in place your chances of quitting for good are even better.

Not all my patients took a drug to help them quit, and not all wanted one. The rare smoker who smokes only a few times a month doesn't usually need a drug to help quit. Most smokers do benefit from medication, without major side effects.

Maybe you worry about medication side effects or getting addicted to medicines. That was Emily's concern. Compared to the side effects of smoking—a shorter, sicker life—taking drugs for a few months to help you quit makes complete sense!

Medicines don't help with the urge to light up after a trigger such as smelling tobacco smoke or seeing an ashtray. They do help with the physical symptoms of withdrawal. That's what Ben told me. They also reduced his desire to smoke. With a milder withdrawal and with less desire to smoke, you'll find it easier to break the habit with new routines that don't include smoking.

All of these medicines are for short-term use, usually about three months. Each one increases your chances of being tobacco-free, and some can be combined for even more benefit. If in an early try to stop smoking you took a medicine that wasn't helpful, try a different one. If you're a very heavy smoker, talk with your doctor about taking two medications instead of one.

A very effective combination of two medications to help with quitting is bupropion, also known as Zyban, and nicotine replacement therapy (using both a patch, for the steady nicotine level, and short-term use of gum when you have a strong urge to smoke). These medications are very helpful if you've had depression or are worried about becoming down or depressed. Another medicine is varenicline, also known by its brand name, Chantix, which you begin taking before you quit.

Once you start a medicine, work closely with your medical team to get help with any side effects or difficulty quitting that you may have. Insurance covers most quit-smoking medications, and co-payments for doctor's office visits will easily be paid for by the money you save by not buying cigarettes. Counseling services and medications are often free through quit lines and are often paid for by public and private insurance plans and clinics.

There is a lot more information about these and other medications in the medication guide section that begins on page 113.

Here's a last thought: twelve weeks of using a drug to help you quit beats twelve more years of smoking.

A cigarette is a poison,
not a reward.

STEP 8
Go cold turkey (and "wild turkey")

THE BEST WAY to quit is to go cold turkey, stopping all at once, but you can ease into the cold turkey phase by first limiting the places you allow yourself to smoke. (I call this going "wild turkey"—I'll explain why in a moment.) Emily and Ben both went cold turkey on the same day. Ben also went wild turkey before his cold turkey day.

Going cold turkey means you can smoke your usual amount of cigarettes until the quit day you've chosen arrives, and then as of that day you're an ex-smoker.

What's "wild turkey"? Turkeys live out in the wild. They don't sit in a comfortable chair in a living room watching TV and having a cigarette. When you go wild turkey, you limit your smoking to one or two places, also out in the wild, where you don't enjoy being. Those places become the only places you allow yourself a cigarette until your chosen quit date a week or two, at most, after going wild turkey. Instead of smoking at home, choose unpleasant places for all your smoking such as standing in your garage, sitting on a park bench a few blocks from home, or standing in the parking lot at work at least a few minutes' walk away from the building.

By not allowing yourself to smoke wherever you wish, you practice controlling smoking urges triggered by situations in which you usually smoke.

Choose a quit date and go cold turkey on that date. If you think going wild turkey with your smoking places beforehand will help, do that too.

*When you quit, smoking
"just one" is like pouring gas
on a fire.*

STEP 9
Toss the smoking tools

GET READY to quit by getting rid of everything in your home, car, and workplace that relates to smoking: matches, lighters, ashtrays, packs, cartons, cigarette cases, holders—even photos on the wall that include a smoker. Clean out your car's ashtray if it has one and remove the lighter. If your car and home smell of tobacco smoke, clean them to remove the smell if you can.

Stock up on sugar-free gum or candies to use as cigarette substitutes and put them in the places you used to keep your cartons, packs, lighters, and matches.

Tell your family and friends that your home and car are now smoke-free zones. Although you'll face triggers elsewhere, cutting out these common triggers makes quitting easier.

Because you've quit the smoking "job," you no longer need the "tools."

To cope with cravings use the Four Ds: delay, deep breaths, drink, and distract.

Step 10
Have a plan for slip-up smoking

ONE OF MY PATIENTS came into my office three months after quitting. I asked him what helped him quit. He told me that when he decided to quit he made up an action plan to use if he thought he was about to slip up. The plan he came up with was this: when he felt the urge to smoke he'd do ten sit-ups or push-ups while singing "Old MacDonald Had a Farm." It didn't matter if he was at home, at work, or driving a car. He'd find a way to do it right away. In the car he'd sing out loud and do sit-ups or push-ups as soon as he got where he was going. At work he explained his behavior to coworkers and went outdoors or into an empty office. Sounds a bit extreme, but it worked for him!

Emily and Ben, like most of my patients, found that taking a few minutes to focus on slow, deep breathing helped them cope with cravings and prevented slip-ups. They did this many times a day, about as often as they used to smoke. It's also a good idea to begin doing this as preparation several times a day for a week or so before your quit date.

Triggers and urges are hard to resist when you're an addict. That's the nature of habit and addiction. Plan to prevent slip-ups, and avoid them at all costs. They just keep the addiction going, like pouring gas on a fire.

If you slip up with one or two smokes, or even a day of smoking, remind yourself of your decision to quit and commit to staying an ex-smoker. You probably were stressed out, on autopilot, or badly in need of a break. Don't waste any energy feeling bad about yourself. It's more important to stay smoke-free. If you've been smoke-free for six months or a year but then smoked for a few days, review what led to your slip-up. Then plan how you could better cope with triggers in the future, contact your quit buddy, and stop immediately. Tell yourself that your period of going smoke-free was a success—on the way to stopping forever—and get back on track.

To resist slip-ups, practice your answers to the following questions:

- How will I respond when a friend offers me a smoke and I really want one?

- The last time I was tempted to smoke, what skills did I use to resist?

- When I'm stressed out, what can I do when I want a smoke?

- What role did my mood, or being around smoking or drinking, play in this slip-up?

Ben and Emily talked through their answers to these questions before they quit. They'd talk about their answers each time before they went out on a Friday or Saturday with friends so they wouldn't slip up.

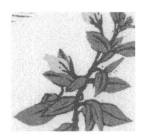

GOLDFISH VINE

3

AFTER
YOU
QUIT

*Having "just one" is how
you became a smoker
in the first place.*

Never buy, bum, or borrow a smoke

ONCE YOU'VE QUIT, you still have a decision to make every day: are you an ex-smoker? This will still be your choice two, five, or ten years later. You'll be at risk of starting up again for many years, so you must stay on guard. Continue to use the four Ds of delay, deep breaths, drink water, and distract. Recognize when your stress level increases; taking steps to lower stress will help you stay smoke-free.

A year after quitting, the usual symptoms of withdrawal are long gone, but you'll still face smoking triggers. They do lessen year by year, but triggers never vanish completely. This isn't your fault—it's because nicotine has changed your brain.

You must renew your decision to be

an ex-smoker every day. Having just one cigarette is how you became a smoker in the first place.

Always refuse any offered cigarette and never borrow, bum, or buy one. Don't test yourself with a smoke. Don't hang around in a smoky place. Don't let down your guard, ever. Why risk a return to smoking?

Tell yourself that you no longer buy, bum, or borrow smokes.

*Not smoking gets easier
with every passing day,
every week, and every month.*

Live strong; live healthy

FEELING DOWN or stressed after quitting is what leads many people to start smoking again. That's what happened to Emily with her earlier quitting efforts. Nicotine affects your brain chemistry. Without it you may feel blue or sad until you recover. When you quit, you can lift your mood by letting go of stress. You could also try bupropion if you're open to taking a medication.

Here are other things you can do:

Just breathe. As a smoker, you took a smoking break each time you lit up. Keep taking the breaks, but consider them breathing breaks, worth celebrating. You took a deep breath in and a long breath out each time you took a drag. Keep doing that but without the smoke. One of the best ways to get past an urge to smoke each time you have one is to do regular breathing. Sit quietly while paying attention only to air flowing in and out through your nose and mouth from your lungs. Do this for at least as long as it usually took you to have a cigarette.[13] Simple meditation or yoga also helps. It's usually easy to find short, free, or low-cost classes where you can learn to do them.

Exercise. Even short, five-minute walks at a slow, medium, or fast pace help when faced with the urge to smoke. A half hour a day or more is best if you can find the time. Any regular exercise that gets you moving works. Exercise helps you cope with low mood and urges to smoke.

Relax. What are your favorite ways to relax? Hobbies, gardening, music, watching TV or playing video games, sports, surfing the web, reading, taking a bath, or being with a nonsmoking friend can all help. It's easy to skip these because of feeling too busy. Your smoking break took time too. Without cigarettes you still need breaks, so make the time. What are your favorite ways to relax other than by smoking?

Think positively. Review the reasons you're doing this difficult thing. Give yourself credit for your hard work and keep at it.

Ben didn't exercise more or take healthy-breathing breaks when he tried to stop before. This time he did both, and he said that it was very helpful for coping with stress and feeling sad.

Remind yourself: "Not smoking gets easier every day, every week, and every month; I can cope without a smoke."

If you quit smoking, others you know may stop too. Children you know may never start.

Celebrate the real rewards

EMILY used the money she saved on tobacco to join a gym. She signed her kids up for an after-school art class. These were her treats for not smoking. Ben bought fishing gear and goes to a nearby lake after work—his reward for quitting.

Early in my work as a doctor in Massachusetts I asked a couple to quit, but I lost track of them because I changed jobs. Years later they saw me in a supermarket, walked up to me with big smiles, thanked me, and said, "Ten years ago you told us to quit. That night we talked about it, quit a week later, and started putting the money we saved on cigarettes into a new bank account. With that money we've been to Alaska, Hawaii, Florida, and Europe. We didn't have money to travel before we quit!"

Reward yourself. Accept the praise you'll get from others for not smoking. If someone you know says something nice about your having quit, don't ignore them. Say, "Thank you for noticing I'm doing well." Pat yourself on the back—you deserve it.

Every month you're smoke-free, do something special as a treat. You can celebrate by telling yourself, "I did well today" or by having a nice dinner or walk with a friend after the first week.

Six months or a year after quitting, treat yourself to a gift, join a health club, take a day off from work, or go on an overnight or weekend vacation.

Do whatever your budget allows that feels special. Create new rewards for having quit.

And if you're asked about quitting by a smoker, tell them how you did it and tell them that if you could do it, they can too. Spread the word: it's not as difficult as many people believe.

Tell yourself: "I don't smoke, because I deserve to be treated well!"

Although you got hooked on smoking, you can become free of your addiction.

Been there, done that. Now I'm doing this!

THERE'S A SAYING that if you don't know where you're going, any road will get you there. You do know where you're going: to being smoke-free, healthy, and strong. Now you've got a road map to get there and the attitude to see you through to the end of that journey. When you have answered yes to the following questions, you are ready to embrace a smoke-free life.

- Do I know why I'm quitting now, and am I ready to do it?

- Do I understand the basics of addiction and withdrawal?

- If I've tried to quit before, do I know what I will do differently this time? Do I know how I will think differently?

- Am I committed to quitting?

Here's your action plan:

- Call a telephone counseling quit line (1-800-QUIT NOW) or join an online group (www.smokefree.gov).

- Find a quit buddy.

- Make a medical appointment to discuss quitting and consider using medications to help quit.

- Choose a date to quit cold turkey; think about going wild turkey too.

- Write a good-bye letter to smoking, then tell everybody you're quitting and ask for support.

- Plan for mood triggers; deal with depression and anxiety.

- Take breathing "celebration breaks," start a half hour of daily walking, stock up on low-calorie snacks and drinks, and plan to relax and keep your hands and mouth busy.

- Stay away from other smokers and cut back on drinking and recreational drug use.

- Know your triggers. Create new routines with new rewards.

- Toss out your smoking tools: lighters, ashtrays, matches, packs, and cartons.

- Have a plan in case you slip up.

- Never buy, borrow, or bum a smoke. Quit for good.

- Stay strong and healthy and celebrate your achievement.

You can overcome your
addiction to smoking.

If you followed the steps and quit

BEST WISHES for your new life as an ex-smoker. I'd like to hear from you. Send me an email at **rbrunswick@ cantquitbullshit.com** or write to me at P.O. Box 1207, Northampton, MA 01061-1207 to let me know how you're doing. I welcome advice on how to improve this book. What was most helpful? What didn't help? What would you like to see added to a future edition?

I may not be able to respond to each email, but I will think about what you say. Thank you for reading this book, and thank you—from my heart—for quitting. I never doubted you could.

—R.B.

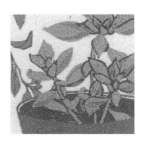

GHOST PLANT

4

USING NICOTINE AND STAYING HEALTHY

Smokeless tobacco may lower health risks by over 90 percent compared with cigarettes.

You can use nicotine, stay healthy, and stop smoking

My HAT'S OFF to you for wanting to quit. I know it's not easy. Not everyone wants to quit. If either Ben or Emily hadn't quit and had asked me, "What should I do next?" here's what I would have told them.

Try again soon. Studies show that most people who do stop have made earlier tries, and that's a good sign of future success at stopping. But there is another way called *the harm-reduction approach*. Instead of smoking to get nicotine, you remain a nicotine addict but don't get it by burning leaf tobacco—i.e., smoking.

What is harm reduction? Just what it sounds like. Driving has accident risks; seat belt use lowers the risk. Drinking and driving has risks; a nondrinking driver lowers the risk. Unsafe sex brings risks of getting illnesses like HIV; condom use lowers the risk. The best harm reduction for nicotine addiction if you can't or don't want to give it up is to find ways to get nicotine into your body other than by smoking tobacco. Nicotine itself isn't a danger except in very high doses; it's the chemicals in tobacco smoke that are dangerous. Here are a few products that deliver nicotine without smoking:

- Nicotine patches, gum, or lozenges.

- Very small, flat, teabag-like pouches, called snuff or snus, that you place under your lip against your gums. They slowly release nicotine.

- Nicotine pellets, wafers, or strips that dissolve in your mouth and slowly release nicotine.

- Electronic cigarettes, known as e-cigs. An e-cigarette is made up of a plastic tube, a tiny container of liquid nicotine, and a heater that releases nicotine as a fine mist without burning it.

All these are ways of taking in nicotine without inhaling the smoke from a burning cigarette. Smokeless tobacco has far fewer chemicals than cigarettes. Newer forms of smokeless tobacco are somewhat like the nicotine gum or patch, but without Food and Drug Administration (FDA) approval. Use one of these not while smoking, but instead of smoking, if you can't quit because of nicotine addiction. None of them causes you to spit out tobacco juice, like the older forms of chewing tobacco.

If you use any of these smoking substitutes, try to cut down and eventually stop using them if you can. If you can't, but you have stopped smoking, you'll be way ahead of the game with regards to health. As long as you don't use them and smoke you will have cut your health risks considerably. Snus, from Sweden, lowers health risks by over 90 percent compared with continuing smoking.[14] It's the chemicals in the smoke, not the nicotine, that cause the health problems from smoking.

Most smokeless tobacco products are already sold in the United States. The small teabag-like pouches or the dissolvable pellets are sold in drugstores, some supermarkets, "big box" stores, online, or in tobacco shops.

Instead of smoking, try one of these products to see what works for you, but note that standard nicotine replacement products like the gum, the patch, and snus products have the most research to show overall safety and benefit. Quit without using them if you can, but use them if you think they'll help.

Here are the details:

• Stay on the nicotine patch, gum, or lozenge long-term. This is probably the safest of the smokeless tobacco choices, if it's what you need to do to quit smoking.

• Try the snus products (the tiny teabag-like sacks) made in Sweden or Denmark. Most Swedish or Danish snus is made with lower levels of some of the harmful chemicals, called nitrosamines (pronounced *nitro-sah-means*), and other additives that are still found at higher levels in some brands made in the United States.

• Use dissolvable nicotine pellets. (Ariva BDL and Stonewall BDL are two brands. Ariva has a lower nicotine content than Stonewall, similar to that of a cigarette.)

• Use an e-cigarette. You buy liquid nicotine for it that comes in different strengths and flavors. Start with one dose of nicotine and gradually lower the strength every three or four weeks if you can. Some research suggests that after cutting down to the lowest level of nicotine, you can use an e-cigarette without any nicotine at all. This is because you'll still have the usual routine of repeated hand-to-mouth smoking activity, and you may not miss the nicotine. I do not recommend any particular brand of e-cigarettes. There is little research at this time that favors one over another and there are some concerns about whether the e-cigarettes and the nicotine substance used with them are being made in ways to keep users safe.[15] Despite this worry, there are many people who have used them to replace smoking, without any problems at all.

You may be wondering whether these products are safe for long-term use. The nicotine patch, gum, or lozenges have not been found to cause diseases such as lung cancer or heart disease. Long-term use of the snus products may very slightly increase the risks of heart attack and cancer of the pancreas, but if so—they cause far, far fewer of these problems than continuing to smoke! Unlike chewing tobacco, they don't cause oral cancers.

Changing from smoking tobacco to long-term use of patches, gum, lozenges, or snus will greatly lower your chances of developing any of those diseases compared with your risks if you continue to smoke. So far, there's not as much research on either the pellets or the e-cigarettes as there is for the nicotine replacement products and snus, so we don't know as much about their safety. If you are considering using any of these other forms of nicotine get your doctor's advice first. They are also likely to be much safer than continuing to smoke.

It would be best if you quit smoking and didn't use these methods. Many smokeless nicotine products, such as snus, are made by big tobacco companies. These companies want what's best for their profits, not what's best for your health. Many public health groups do not approve of smokeless sources of nicotine even as they accept that a person who uses a smokeless form of nicotine, instead of smoking, stands to gain a lot, health-wise. Their main concern is that minors who are tempted to try smokeless forms of nicotine might be tempted to try cigarettes as well. For that reason, I recommend smokeless nicotine products only to smokers who seek a much safer alternative to smoking.

Because nicotine is a drug, whether prescribed or not, talk to your doctor about using these forms of nicotine before you start them. Many doctors don't know about these alternatives to smoking. You'll find more information on smokeless tobacco on page 133. You can read and share it with your doctor.

If you stop smoking by using one of the smokeless ways to get nicotine, I'd like to hear from you about your experience. Send me an email at **rbrunswick@cantquit-bullshit.com** or write to me at P.O. Box 1207, Northampton, MA 01061-1207 with advice about how I could improve this book. Thank you for reading it.

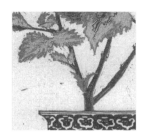

COLEUS

5

RESOURCES

Spread the word: once you've quit, let others know they can stop too.

Support

MANY different groups (health insurers, employers, organizations, state public health departments, hospitals, and others) offer help for people who want to stop smoking. Here's what I suggest you do to find out about what's available to you.

1. Ask your doctor, your local hospital, and the local or state public health department about any programs in your area to help smokers.

2. Check with national groups such as the American Cancer Society or the American Lung Association about services they offer, whether web-based, phone-based, or with individual or group counseling. There are programs in many languages. Your local librarian can also be of help.

3. If you have health insurance, ask the insurer whether stop-smoking support or counseling and stop-smoking medicines (such as the nicotine patch, which doesn't require a prescription) are covered by the plan. Have them send you the details about the coverage. You will want to know what they pay, what you have to pay, and what type of support and which drugs they cover.

4. I advise visiting several websites to find needed help. My favorites are Smokefree.gov (www.smokefree.gov) and its companion site just for women (www.women.smokefree.gov).

Quit-smoking Contacts

NAME: American Cancer Society
PHONE: 800-227-2345
WEB: www.cancer.org
NOTES: Click on "Stay Healthy," then "Stay Away from Tobacco"; see also "Quit for Life"

NAME: American Heart Association
PHONE: 800-242-8721
WEB: www.heart.org
NOTES: Eng., Span., Vietnamese, Chinese

NAME: American Legacy Foundation Quitline
PHONE: 202-454-5555
WEB: www.legacyforhealth.org
www.becomeanex.org
NOTES: Eng., Span., and services for pregnant smokers

NAME: American Lung Association
PHONE: 800-548-8252
WEB: www.lung.org
NOTES: Eng., Span.; click on "Stop Smoking" or use this address: www.lung.org/stop-smoking

NAME: National Cancer Institute Quitline
PHONE: 877-448-7848
WEB: www.smokefree.gov
www.women.smokefree.gov
NOTES: Eng., Span.; live help Mon.–Fri., 8 a.m. to 8 p.m. EST

NAME: National Institute of Drug Abuse
PHONE: 800-784-8669
         301-443-1124 (English)
         240-221-4007 (Spanish)
WEB: www.nida.nih.gov
NOTES: Eng., Span.

NAME: National Network of Tobacco
         Cessation Quitlines
PHONE: 800-784-8669
WEB: smokefree.gov/expert.aspx
NOTES: Eng., Span.

NAME: National Spit Tobacco
         Education Project
PHONE: 312-836-9900
WEB: oralhealthamerica.org/programs/nstep
NOTES: Eng., Span., Vietnamese, Chinese

NAME: Nicotine Anonymous
PHONE: 877-879-6422
WEB: www.nicotine-anonymous.org
NOTES: Eng., Span., Vietnamese, Chinese

*Using medications to help
quit doubles the chance that
you'll really stop.*

Drugs that help you quit

T HE FOLLOWING INFORMATION comes from
Smokefree.gov (www.smokefree.gov),
a website of the National Cancer Institute,
a government agency. I've shortened it to
the basics for each medicine, including
how to use it, dosing, side effects, and
warnings. If you prefer, you can go to
Smokefree.gov's medication guide and
click directly on the link for each medication's fact sheet. After the guide and fact
sheets I've added my thoughts about each
of the three most commonly used medications: **nicotine replacement therapy**,
bupropion (Zyban), and **varenicline
(Chantix)**. Before using any medications,
discuss them with your physician.

Those who get help with quitting are the most likely to stop and be smoke-free one year after stopping.

Medication guide

THIS GUIDE reviews the current medications used by smokers who are trying to quit. It may not include every medication available. All of these medications have been shown to be useful for helping smokers quit. No one medication works best for all smokers. Always read the instructions on the package carefully and talk with your doctor or pharmacist if you have questions. The dosing information is meant only to show how most people use these medications. The dose of your prescription medications must be decided by a doctor. If you are pregnant, breast-feeding, or have a severe medical problem, talk with your doctor before starting any new medication.

First-line Medications: Nicotine Replacement Therapy (NRT)

These medications are called "first-line" because many smokers use these when they first try to quit. If the first-line medications don't work, smokers might try a second-line medication instead.

Nicotine replacement therapy (NRT) helps smokers quit by reducing their craving sensations. These craving sensations happen when the body goes through withdrawal from the nicotine in tobacco. NRT products provide controlled amounts of nicotine. Individuals reduce their use of NRT products over time, allowing their bodies to gradually adjust to decreasing nicotine levels.

Nicotine patches (over the counter)

The nicotine patch, placed on the skin, supplies a small and steady amount of nicotine to the body. Nicotine patches contain varied amounts of nicotine (21 milligrams [mg], 14mg, or 7mg, for example), and the user reduces the dose over time. (smoke free.gov/mg-nicotine_patch.aspx)

Nicotine gum (over the counter)

Nicotine gum is chewed to release nicotine inside the mouth. The user chews the gum until it produces a tingling feeling, then places (parks) it between the cheek and gum tissue. Nicotine gums have varied amounts of nicotine (typically 2mg or 4mg) to allow users to reduce the amount of nicotine in their bodies. (smokefree.gov /mg-nicotine_gum.aspx)

Nicotine lozenges (over the counter)

Nicotine lozenges look like hard candy. The lozenges (typically containing a 2-mg or 4-mg dose of nicotine) release nicotine as they slowly dissolve in the mouth. (smoke free.gov/mg-nicotine_lozenges.aspx)

Nicotine inhaler (prescription)

A nicotine inhaler is a cartridge attached to a mouthpiece. Inhaling through the mouthpiece delivers a specific amount of nicotine to the user. (smokefree.gov/mg-nicotine_inhaler.aspx)

Nicotine nasal spray (prescription)

Nicotine nasal spray comes in a pump bottle, the tip of which is inserted into the nose and sprayed. Nicotine nasal spray can be used for immediate craving control, especially for heavy smokers. (smokefree .gov/mg-nicotine_spray.aspx)

OTHER FIRST-LINE MEDICATIONS

Bupropion (prescription)

Bupropion, also known as Zyban, helps to reduce nicotine withdrawal symptoms and the urge to smoke. Bupropion can be used safely with nicotine replacement products. (smokefree.gov/mg-bupropion.aspx)

Varenicline (prescription)

Varenicline, also known as Chantix, is a prescription medication that eases nicotine withdrawal symptoms and blocks the effects of nicotine from cigarettes if the user starts smoking again. (smokefree.gov /mg-varenicline.aspx)

References: Information in the medication guide and fact sheets comes from a variety of sources, such as product information guides, manufacturers' websites, medical websites, and articles in the medical literature, including Corelli, R. L. and Hudman, K. S., "Pharmacologic interventions for smoking cessation," *Critical Care Nursing Clinics of North America* 2006; pp. 18, 39–51.

Drug Fact Sheets

These general precautions apply to each fact sheet:

The fact sheets were created to give you a general understanding of these medications. Please note that they may not provide you with all the information you need to make a decision about using these medications. Always read the instructions on the package carefully and talk with your doctor or pharmacist if you have questions. If you are pregnant, breast-feeding, or have a severe medical problem, talk with your doctor before starting any new medication.

NICOTINE PATCH FACT SHEET

The nicotine patch is placed on the skin and supplies a small and steady amount of nicotine into the body. Nicotine patches contain varied amounts of nicotine (21mg, 14mg, or 7mg, for example), and the user reduces the dose over time. Available in generic forms and under the brand names Nicotrol, Nicoderm CQ.

Dosing

For individuals who smoke more than 10 cigarettes/day:

Nicotrol: 15-mg/day for 6 weeks, then 10-mg/day for 2 weeks, then 5-mg/day for 2 weeks.

Nicoderm CQ: 21-mg/day for 6 weeks, then 14-mg/day for 2 weeks, then 7-mg/day for 2 weeks.

Generic: 21-mg/day for 6 weeks, then 14-mg/day for 2 weeks, then 7-mg/day for 2 weeks.

For individuals who smoke 10 or fewer cigarettes/day:

Nicotrol: Not recommended.

Nicoderm CQ: 14-mg/day for 6 weeks, then 7-mg/day for 2 weeks.

Generic: 14-mg/day for 6 weeks, then 7-mg/day for 2 weeks.

Side effects

- Headaches
- Dizziness/lightheadedness
- Drowsiness
- Upset stomach/nausea

Special precautions

Pregnancy/breast-feeding: Smokers who

are pregnant or breast-feeding should try to quit without using the nicotine patch. The nicotine patch should be used during pregnancy only if the associated benefits outweigh the associated risks.

Heart conditions: Smokers who have serious arrhythmias or have chest pains due to coronary artery disease should use the nicotine patch with caution.

Skin conditions: Smokers who have skin disorders (e.g., psoriasis, eczema, or atopic dermatitis) may experience skin irritation.

NICOTINE GUM FACT SHEET

Nicotine gum is chewed to release nicotine inside the mouth. The user chews the gum until it produces a tingling feeling, then the gum is placed (parked) between the cheek and gum tissue. Nicotine gums have varied amounts of nicotine (typically 2mg or 4mg) to allow users to reduce the amount of nicotine in their bodies.

Dosing

For individuals smoking 25 or more cigarettes a day: 4-mg.

For individuals smoking fewer than 25 cigarettes a day: 2-mg.

Weeks 1–6: one piece every 1 to 2 hrs.

Weeks 7–9: one piece every 2 to 4 hrs.

Weeks 10–12: one piece every 4 to 8 hrs.

Side effects
- A bad taste from the gum
- Tingling feeling on tongue when chewing gum
- Hiccups
- Upset stomach and/or nausea
- Heartburn
- Jaw pain caused by chewing

Special precautions

Pregnancy/breast-feeding: Smokers who are pregnant or breast-feeding should try to quit first without using the nicotine gum. Nicotine gum should be used during pregnancy only if the associated benefits outweigh the associated risks.

Temporomandibular joint (TMJ) pain (jaw pain): Nicotine gum may not be appropriate for smokers who have been diagnosed with TMJ or have bridges or dentures.

NICOTINE LOZENGES FACT SHEET

Nicotine lozenges look like hard candy. The lozenges (typically containing a 2-mg or 4-mg dose of nicotine) release nicotine as they slowly dissolve in the mouth.

Dosing
For individuals who smoke their first cigarette 30 minutes after waking up or sooner: 4-mg.

For individuals who smoke their first cigarette more than 30 minutes after waking up: 2 -mg.

Weeks 1–6: one lozenge every 1 to 2 hrs.

Weeks 7–9: one lozenge every 2 to 4 hrs.

Weeks 10–12: one lozenge every 4 to 8 hrs.

Side effects
- Soreness of teeth and gums
- Indigestion
- Irritated throat

Special precautions
Pregnancy/breast-feeding: Smokers who

are pregnant or breast-feeding should try to quit first without using the nicotine lozenges. The nicotine lozenge should be used during pregnancy only if the associated benefits outweigh the associated risks.

Heart conditions: Smokers who have serious arrhythmias or have chest pains due to coronary artery disease should use the nicotine lozenge with caution.

NICOTINE INHALER FACT SHEET

A nicotine inhaler is a cartridge attached to a mouthpiece. Inhaling through the mouthpiece delivers a set amount of nicotine to the user.

Dosing

Six to 16 cartridges daily (approximately one cartridge every 1 to 2 hours). Each cartridge delivers 4-mg of nicotine over 80 to 100 inhalations (approximately 20 minutes of active puffing). Recommended duration of therapy is up to 6 months (decrease dosage during last 3 months of treatment).

Side effects
- Throat irritation
- Mouth irritation
- Coughing

Special precautions
Pregnancy/breast-feeding: Smokers who are pregnant or breast-feeding should try to quit first without using the nicotine inhaler. The nicotine inhaler should be used during pregnancy only if the associated benefits outweigh the associated risks.

Breathing conditions: Smokers with lung problems, such as asthma, should use the nicotine inhaler with caution.

NICOTINE NASAL SPRAY FACT SHEET

Nicotine nasal spray comes in a pump bottle, the tip of which is inserted into the nose and sprayed. Nicotine nasal spray can be used for immediate craving control, especially for heavy smokers.

Dosing
One to 2 sprays in each nostril per hour. Increase as needed for symptom relief. Recommended duration of therapy: 3–6 months.

Side effects
- Sneezing
- Coughing
- Watering eyes

Special precautions

Pregnancy/breast-feeding: Smokers who are pregnant or breast-feeding should try to quit first without using the nicotine nasal spray. The nicotine nasal spray should be used during pregnancy only if the associated benefits outweigh the associated risks.

Chronic nose/lung conditions: Smokers with chronic nasal disorders (e.g., rhinitis, polyps, sinusitis) or those who have severe reactive airway disease should not use the nicotine nasal spray.

Dependence: The nicotine nasal spray may be addicting, and individuals may find that the dependence is more than with other nicotine replacement therapy products.

BUPROPION FACT SHEET

Bupropion, also known as Zyban, helps to reduce nicotine withdrawal symptoms and the urge to smoke. Bupropion can be used safely with nicotine replacement products.

Dosing

Take 150-mg every morning for 3 days. Then increase to 150 -mg twice daily for 7 to 12 weeks. Unlike nicotine replacement therapy products, smokers should begin treatment with bupropion 1 to 2 weeks before they quit smoking. For maintenance therapy, smokers can take 150-mg twice daily for up to 6 months.

Side effects

- Dry mouth
- Difficulty sleeping
- Headaches
- Dizziness
- Skin rashes

Special precautions

Pregnancy/breast-feeding: Smokers who are pregnant or breast-feeding should try to quit first without using bupropion. Bupropion should be used during pregnancy only if the associated benefits outweigh the associated risks.

Seizures: Smokers who have a history of seizures, cranial trauma, or severe liver impairment must use bupropion with extreme caution.

VARENICLINE FACT SHEET

Varenicline, also known as Chantix, is a prescription medication that eases nicotine withdrawal symptoms and blocks the effects of nicotine from cigarettes if the user starts smoking again.

Dosing
One pill twice daily.

Side effects
- Nausea
- Change in dreaming
- Constipation
- Gas
- Vomiting

There have been rare reports of mood swings, depression, and suicidal thoughts. Your doctor will want to monitor this carefully. Please check the FDA website (www.fda.gov) for updates about this medication.

Special precautions
Pregnancy/breastfeeding: Smokers who are pregnant or breastfeeding should try to quit first without using varenicline. Varenicline should be used during pregnancy

only if the associated benefits outweigh the associated risks.

Kidney problems: Smokers should not use varenicline if they have kidney problems.

More on Medicines to Help You Quit

I believe smokers should go cold turkey instead of gradually cutting down after preparing for quitting. I also believe it's a good idea to use a medication as long as you understand its pros and cons and how to use it.

Nicotine replacement therapy (NRT)

Nicotine replacement is called "replacement" for a reason: you're supposed to use it instead of smoking, not along with smoking. Using them together just keeps you an addict. Don't do it.

All NRTs get nicotine to the brain more slowly than smoking. All cut down urges. Since you also need to learn to deal with triggers and change your routines, replacing nicotine to cut down withdrawal gives you a chance to work on two problems instead of three: you can deal with triggers and learn new routines without urges.

A common mistake when trying nicotine replacement is to not use the right dose. The 21-mg patch gives you about the same amount of nicotine you'd find in a pack of cigarettes. The 14-mg patch is equal to 14 cigarettes, and the 7-mg patch is equal to about 7 cigarettes.

If you smoke two packs (40 cigarettes) a day, you might try two 21-mg patches, equal to 42-mg a day. This adds expense; other experts say one patch is enough even if you smoke more than a pack a day. While the patches come with overdose warnings, and you should be familiar with the symptoms, like nausea and dizziness, this isn't usually a problem.[16] Discuss this with your doctor first.

Research shows that if you begin using a nicotine patch two weeks before your quit date you'll have an easier time of quitting permanently.[17]

Lots of smokers use nicotine gum. Like the patch, it's available without a prescription. It comes in two strengths, 2-mg and 4-mg per piece. Similar to smoking, it keeps your mouth busy. You chew it a bit, park the gum in your cheek, and give the gum a few chews every few minutes to release more nicotine. The gum and the lozenges need replacing regularly, while the patch is applied once a day and provides a steadier level of nicotine.

The patch and gum or lozenge can be used together. As urges are often strongest upon awakening, when patch nicotine levels are at their lowest, I tell smokers using patches to try nicotine gum or lozenges first thing in the morning and for a few hours afterward until the new patch gets the nicotine level back up. Use the gum upon awakening each day rather than waiting for an urge to smoke. You can use up to sixteen pieces a day; they work best if you use a new one every hour or two. After several weeks you can try to stop the gum and just continue with the patch. Don't use more than is recommended.

I don't advise either nicotine nasal spray or inhalers. They seem to have more side effects, cost more than the gum or patch, and require frequent use, but if either appeals to you, try it instead of the other forms.

In January 2012, a new research study raised doubts about NRT's effectiveness,[18] but the new study's findings have been challenged.[19] It's been known for a long time that NRT won't quit for you, but combined with support or counseling and a motivated quitter, most studies show that NRT is of real benefit for quitting.

Bupropion (also known as **Zyban**, and by other names)

Bupropion is sold as a generic drug that's usually less expensive than Zyban. From here on, I will only refer to bupropion (pronounced *boo-pro-pea-on*). You need a prescription to get it.

Bupropion was first developed to treat depression. It doesn't contain or replace nicotine. People taking it find that it really helps them quit smoking by lowering their urges to smoke and damping the pleasure they get from smoking. This makes withdrawal easier. It helps smokers who are and aren't depressed. It can help with the down mood that often develops when quitting, even if you don't have full-blown depression.

Like nicotine replacement, it doubles the quit rate compared to those who try without medications.

If you're concerned about either weight gain or low mood when quitting, bupropion is a better choice than nicotine replacement as it helps with both in addition to lowering the urge to smoke. Many people use bupropion and nicotine replacement together, but this adds cost and increases the risk of side effects. If you've tried to quit with one or the other and couldn't, you could try both.

Varenicline (also known as **Chantix**)

Chantix is the newest quitting drug. It has mild nicotine-like effects on the brain even though it isn't nicotine. It cuts smoking pleasure and the urge to smoke.

You take it once a day to start for a few days then twice a day as you increase the dose. It can cause suicidal thoughts and behaviors, agitation, hostility, and other side effects. It may increase the risk of a heart attack, so you should talk about it with your doctor. Ex-smokers who've used varenicline have a somewhat better rate of staying tobacco-free than those who've used bupropion or nicotine replacement, but the drug is more expensive than other options.

You can *stop smoking.*

Lowering Tobacco's Harm: More Information

YOU CAN GET more information on harm reduction to lower the health risks from smoking. Using smokeless tobacco products to cut harm is a somewhat new area of study, and there's more to learn.

The best review of this topic was carried out by the Royal College of Physicians' Tobacco Advisory Group in 2007.[20] The Royal College of Physicians is a very highly regarded group in England that began in 1518 and is devoted to improving healthcare and the practice of medicine in the United Kingdom. The report is very complete and includes many references. You can read the full report or just the conclusions at the end of each section if you prefer. You'll find the report at www.rcplondon.ac.uk. To read it, click on

"Resources," then, under "Bookshop," click on "Browse the bookshop," then click on "Publications by Title," and then "Harm Reduction in Nicotine Addiction: Helping People Who Can't Quit." It may be ordered as a book for a fee or downloaded for free.

The American Association of Public Health Physicians website has lots of information on harm reduction and smoking; the address is www.aaphp.org. First click on "General Resources," then "Tobacco." You can read and print the information directly from the website. It includes links to articles on this topic.

A very good summary about smokeless tobacco can be found in the journal Tobacco Control. The article is: "Noncigarette tobacco products: what have we learnt and where are we headed?" by Richard J. O'Connor. You can read it, or get it at: http://tobaccocontrol.bmj.com/content/21/2/181.abstract. Then click on "full text" on the right side. It has good information on the pros and cons of using them.

If you don't have a computer or need help finding this material, your public library staff can help.

Endnotes

[1] Charles Duhigg, *The Power of Habit* (New York: Random House; 2012), p. 19.

[2] Duhigg, p. 25.

[3] Kenneth Perkins et al., *Cognitive Behavioral Therapy for Smoking Cessation* (New York: Routledge; 2008), p. 168.

[4] Perkins, pp. 172–178.

[5] Jonathan Diamond, *Narrative Means to Sober Ends* (New York: Guilford Press; 2000), p. 33.

[6] Deborah Ritchie et al., *The "Smokey Joe Story" Handbook: A Micro Analysis of the "Smokey Joe" Smoking Cessation* (Scotland: ASH; 2005), pp. 63–155.

[7] Somov et al., *The Smoke-Free Smoke Break* (Oakland: New Harbinger; 2011), p. 46.

[8] Somov et al., p. 41.

[9] Daniel Seidman, *Smoke-Free in 30 Days* (New York: Simon and Schuster; 2010), p. 95.

[10] makesmokinghistory.org/quitting/steps-to-help-you-quit/two/be-ready-for-challenges.html (accessed on 9.19.12).

[11] Duhigg, p. 78.

[12] Perkins, pp. 63, 76–78.

[13] Somov et al., p. 154.

14 "Harm reduction in nicotine addiction: Helping people who can't quit." (Royal College of Physicians, London: Royal College of Physicians; 2007), pp. 130–131. www.tobaccoprogram.org/pdf/4fc74817-64c5-4105-951e-38239b09c5db.pdf (accessed on 8.26.12).

15 "Non-cigarette tobacco products: what have we learnt and where are we headed?" (O'Connor, R.J.; Tobacco Control; 2012:21 181-190). http://tobaccocontrol.bmj.com/content/21/2/181.abstract. (Accessed on 10.9.12.) doi:10.1136/tobaccocontrol-2011-050281.

16 Seidman, pp. 50–51, 62.

17 Seidman, pp. 76–77.

18 "A prospective cohort study challenging the effectiveness of population-based medical intervention for smoking cessation" (Alpert, H. R., Connolly, G. N., and Biener, L.; http://www.ncbi.nlm.nih.gov/pubmed/22234781?dopt=Abstract

19 Statement by the Association for the Treatment of Tobacco Use and Dependence (ATTUD) regarding "A prospective cohort study challenging the effectiveness of population-based medical intervention for smoking cessation" (Alpert, H. R., Connolly, G. N., and Biener, L.; *Tobacco Control;* January 10, 2012); www.attud.org/pdf/ATTUD_statement2012.pdf (accessed on 8.26.12).

20 "Harm reduction in nicotine addiction: Helping people who can't quit." (see note 14).

Acknowledgments

Many people helped with this book. My friends gave invaluable advice: Marci Yoss, Elizabeth Erickson, Barry Feingold, David Greenberg, David Kittay, Don Lehn, Deborah Schifter, Louise Dejardins, and Henry Simkin.

Family members provided great support and advice: Elena and Lilly Betke-Brunswick, Jamie Sweeney, William and Margaret Betke, Barbara and Noah Suddaby, and Roger, Fred, and Hilde Brunswick. I received valuable assistance from Dr. C. Tracy Orleans and Dr. Kenneth Michael Cummings.

Hans Teensma provided book design services and encouragement, and Elena Betke-Brunswick provided artwork. My editors, Carolyn Edelstein, Jean Zimmer, and Gregory Lauzon, made this book possible, and I am grateful for their excellent assistance.

This book is dedicated to my patients, who bravely spoke of their addiction to tobacco, and to my late wife, Elizabeth Betke.

NOTES

NOTES

NOTES

NOTES

Pass this book around.
Give a copy to family, friends,
co-workers — anyone you want
to help kick the habit.
Can't Quit? Bullsh*t! is also available
from: www.cantquitbullshit.com
where you'll find useful information
and a link to the author's e-store
for secure, fast ordering.